Diabetic Diet Cookbook for Your Lunch & Dinner

A Collection of Delicious Diabetic Recipes for Your Daily Meals

Roseann Smith

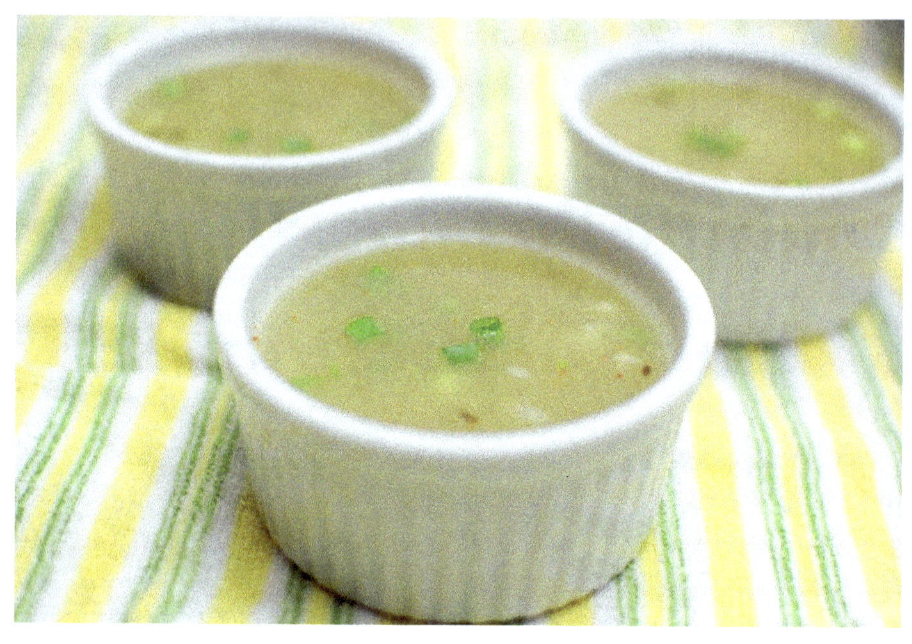

Disclaimer Notice:

Please note the information contained within this document is for educational and entertainment purposes only. All effort has been executed to present accurate, up to date, and reliable, complete information. No warranties of any kind are declared or implied. Readers acknowledge that the author is not engaging in the rendering of legal, financial, medical or professional advice. The content within this book has been derived from various sources. Please consult a licensed professional before attempting any techniques outlined in this book.

By reading this document, the reader agrees that under no circumstances is the author responsible for any losses, direct or indirect, which are incurred as a result of the use of information contained within this document, including, but not limited to, — errors, omissions, or inaccuracies.

Table of Contents

Salmon With Pineapple-cilantro Salsa

Servings: 4

Cooking Time: 15 Minutes

Ingredients:

- 1 lb. salmon fillets, skinless, 1 inch thick
- 2 tablespoons parsley or cilantro, chopped
- 2 cups pineapple, chopped
- ¼ cup red onion, chopped
- ½ cup green or red bell pepper, chopped
- What you will need from the store cupboard:
- ¼ teaspoon salt
- ½ teaspoon chili powder
- 3 tablespoons lime juice
- Lime wedges, optional
- Pinch of cayenne pepper

Directions:

1. Rinse the fish. Use paper towels to pat dry.

2. For the salsa, bring together the bell pepper, pineapple, lime juice, red onion, and a tablespoon of parsley or cilantro in a bowl. Keep this aside.

3. Now combine the lime juice, salt, and the remaining parsley or cilantro.

4. Brush this on both sides of your fish.

5. Keep fish on your grill and grill for 8 minutes. Turn once.

6. Cut your fish into 4 serving sizes. Apply salsa on top.

7. You can serve with lettuce and lime wedges.

Nutrition Info: Calories 257, Carbohydrates 13g, Fiber 2g, Sugar 1g, Cholesterol 66mg, Total Fat 12g, Protein 23g

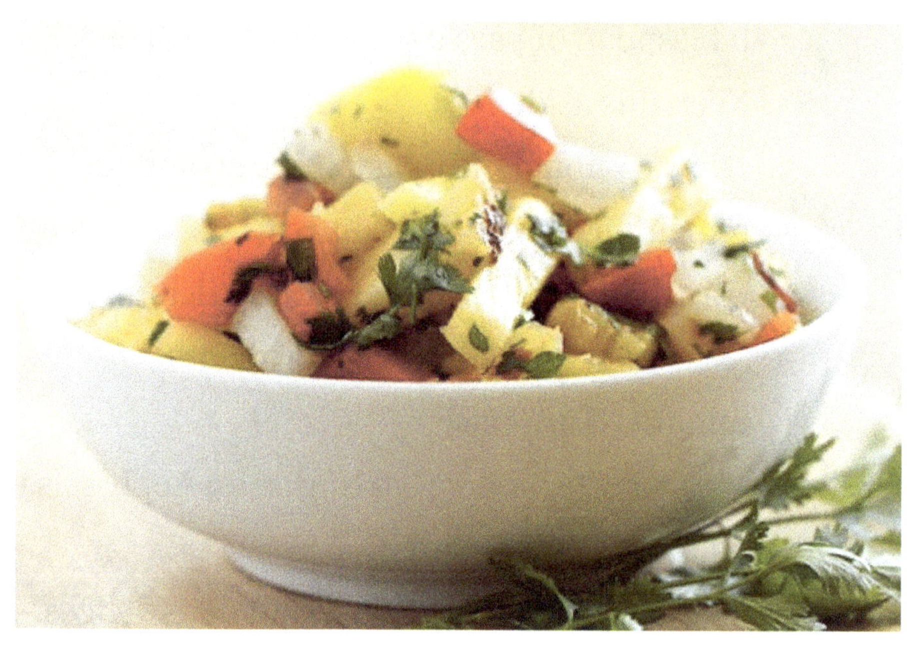

Italian Tuna Pasta

Servings: 6

Cooking Time: 5 Minutes

Ingredients:

- 15 oz whole wheat pasta
- 2 tbsp capers
- 3 oz tuna
- 2 cups can tomatoes, crushed
- 2 anchovies
- 1 tsp garlic, minced
- 1 tbsp olive oil
- Salt

Directions:

1. Add oil into the inner pot of instant pot and set the pot on sauté mode.
2. Add anchovies and garlic and sauté for 1 minute.

3. Add remaining ingredients and stir well. Pour enough water into the pot to cover the pasta.

4. Seal pot with a lid and select manual and cook on low for 4 minutes.

5. Once done, release pressure using quick release. Remove lid.

6. Stir and serve.

Nutrition Info: Calories 339 Fat 6 g Carbohydrates 56.5 g Sugar 5.2 g Protein 15.2 g Cholesterol 10 mg

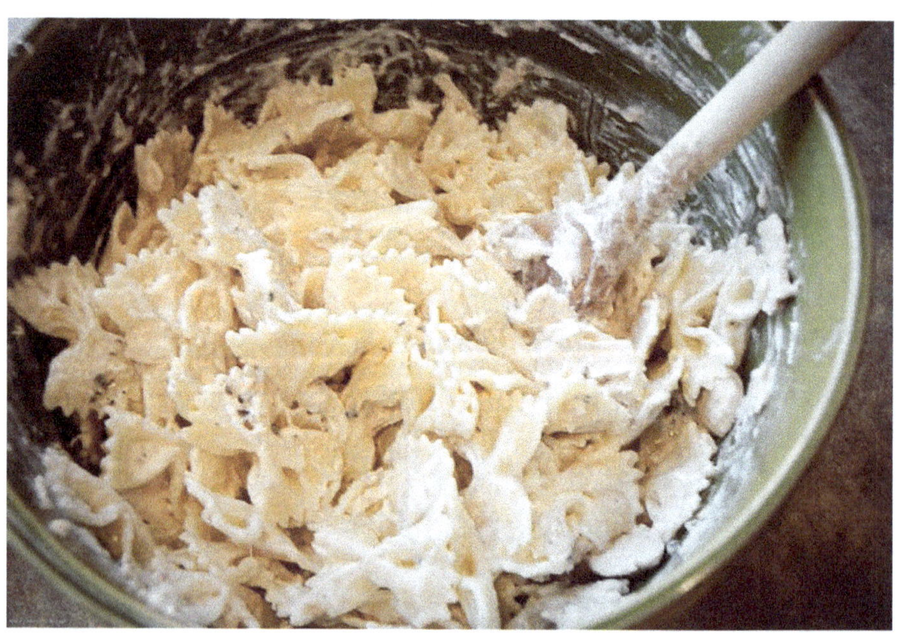

Baked Salmon With Garlic Parmesan Topping

Servings: 4

Cooking Time: 20 Minutes,

Ingredients:

- 1 lb. wild caught salmon filets
- 2 tbsp. margarine
- What you'll need from store cupboard:
- ¼ cup reduced fat parmesan cheese, grated
- ¼ cup light mayonnaise
- 2-3 cloves garlic, diced
- 2 tbsp. parsley
- Salt and pepper

Directions:

1. Heat oven to 350 and line a baking pan with parchment paper.
2. Place salmon on pan and season with salt and pepper.

3. In a medium skillet, over medium heat, melt butter. Add garlic and cook, stirring 1 minute.

4. Reduce heat to low and add remaining Ingredients. Stir until everything is melted and combined.

5. Spread evenly over salmon and bake 15 minutes for thawed fish or 20 for frozen. Salmon is done when it flakes easily with a fork. Serve.

Nutrition Info: Calories 408 Total Carbs 4g Protein 41g Fat 24g Sugar 1g Fiber 0g

Cucumber Salad With Pesto

Servings: 4

Cooking Time: 0 Minute

Ingredients:

- 1 cup fresh basil leaves, chopped
- 2 cloves garlic
- 2 tablespoons walnuts
- 1 teaspoon Parmesan cheese
- 1 tablespoon olive oil
- 2 cucumbers, sliced into rounds
- Salt and pepper to taste

Directions:

1. Put the basil, garlic, walnuts, Parmesan cheese and olive oil in a food processor.
2. Pulse until smooth.
3. Season the cucumbers with salt and pepper.
4. Spread pesto on top of each cucumber round.

Nutrition Info: Calories 80 Total Fat 6g Saturated Fat 0.7g Cholesterol 0mg Sodium 4mg Total Carbohydrate 6.5g Dietary Fiber 1.2g Total Sugars 2.6g Protein 2.2g Potassium 266mg

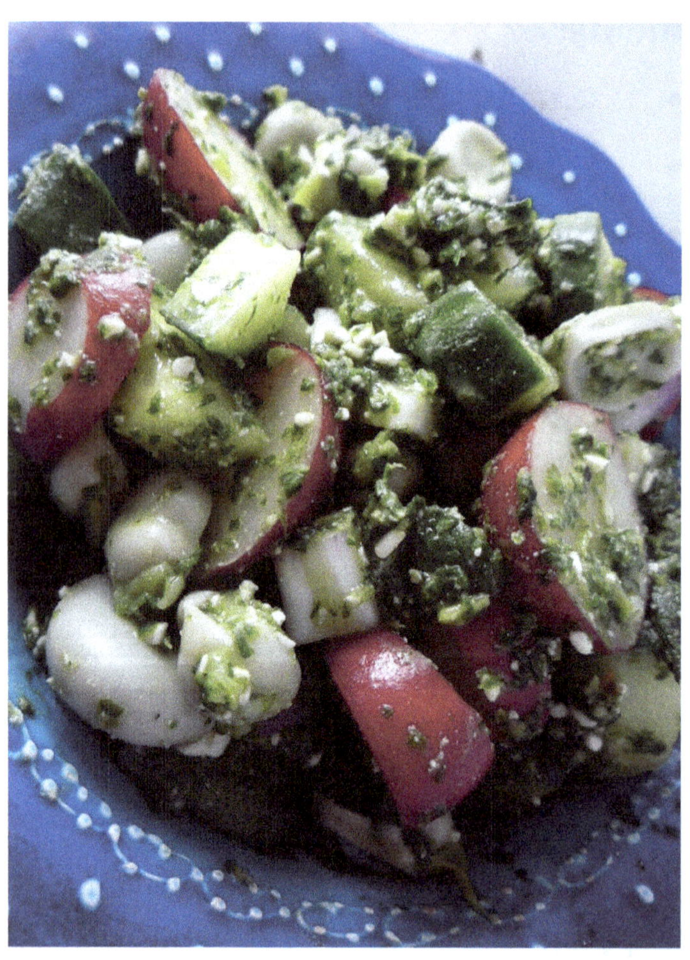

Easy Brussels Sprouts Hash

Servings: 4

Cooking Time: 10 Minutes

Ingredients:

- 3 tablespoons extra-virgin olive oil
- 1 onion, finely chopped
- 1 pound Brussels sprouts, bottoms trimmed off, shredded (see tip)
- ½ teaspoon caraway seeds
- ½ teaspoon sea salt
- ⅛ teaspoon freshly ground black pepper
- ¼ cup red wine vinegar
- 1 tablespoon Dijon mustard
- 1 tablespoon honey
- 3 garlic cloves, minced

Directions:

1. In a large skillet over medium-high heat, heat the olive oil until it shimmers.

2. Add the onion, Brussels sprouts, caraway seeds, sea salt, and pepper. Cook for 7 to 10 minutes, stirring occasionally, until the Brussels sprouts begin to brown.

3. While the Brussels sprouts cook, whisk the vinegar, mustard, and honey in a small bowl and set aside.

4. Add the garlic to the skillet and cook for 30 seconds, stirring constantly.

5. Add the vinegar mixture to the skillet. Cook for about 5 minutes, stirring, until the liquid reduces by half.

Nutrition Info: Calories: 176; Protein: 11g; Total Carbohydrates: 19g; Sugars: 8g; Fiber: 5g; Total Fat: 11g; Saturated Fat: 1g; Cholesterol: 0mg; Sodium: 309mg

Vegetable And Bean Stew

Servings: 6

Cooking Time: 20 Minutes

Ingredients:

- 1 lb. potatoes, cut into small 1 inch chunks
- 2 parsnips, 1-inch chunks
- 2 carrots, 1-inch chunks
- 19 oz. pinto beans, drained and rinsed
- 1 acorn squash
- What you will need from the store cupboard:
- 2 teaspoons olive oil
- 1 cup apple cider
- 1 cup vegetable broth, low-sodium
- Salt and pepper to taste

Directions:

1. Preheat your oven to 350 °F.
2. Divide the squash. Remove the seeds. Cut the flesh into 4 cm chunks and peel the skin.

3. Put them in a bowl and also the carrots, potatoes, and parsnips.
4. Drizzle olive oil. Toss well to coat.
5. Now stir the garlic in. Season with pepper and salt lightly.
6. Keep the rosemary sprigs in your roasting pan.
7. Spread vegetables in a single layer on top.
8. Roast to brown lightly. Turn once.
9. Take out from the oven. Stir the cider, broth and pinto beans in.
10. Use foil to cover your pan tightly.
11. Cook until your vegetables have become tender.
12. Garnish with rosemary sprigs.

Nutrition Info: Calories 278, Fat 3g, Protein 8g, Carbohydrates 58g, Fiber 11g, Cholesterol 0mg, Sugar 0.6g

Grilled Zucchini With Tomato Relish

Servings: 4

Cooking Time: 10 Minutes

Ingredients:

- 1 lb. zucchini, sliced in half
- 1 tablespoon olive oil
- Salt and pepper to taste
- 1 teaspoon red wine vinegar
- 1 tablespoon mint, chopped
- 1 cup tomatoes, chopped

Directions:

1. Preheat your grill.
2. Brush both sides of zucchini with oil and season with salt and pepper.
3. Grill for 3 to 4 minutes per side.
4. In a bowl, mix the rest of the ingredients with the remaining oil.
5. Season with salt and pepper.

6. Spread tomato relish on top of the grilled zucchini before serving.

Nutrition Info: Calories 71 Total Fat 5 g Saturated Fat 1 g Cholesterol 0 mg Sodium 157 mg Total Carbohydrate 6 g Dietary Fiber 2 g Total Sugars 4 g Protein 2 g Potassium 413 mg

Carrot Soup With Tempeh

Servings: 6

Cooking Time: 45 Minutes

Ingredients:

- ¼ cup olive oil, divided
- 1 large yellow onion, chopped
- Salt, to taste
- 2 pounds' carrots, peeled, and cut into ½-inch rounds
- 2 tablespoons fresh dill, chopped
- 4½ cups homemade vegetable broth
- 12 ounces' tempeh, cut into ½-inch cubes
- ¼ cup tomato paste
- 1 teaspoon fresh lemon juice

Directions:

1. In a large soup pan, heat 2 tablespoons of the oil over medium heat and cook the onion with salt for about 6–8 minutes, stirring frequently.

2. Add the carrots and stir to combine.

3. Lower the heat to low and cook, covered for about 5 minutes, stirring frequently.

4. Add in the broth and bring to a boil over high heat.

5. Lower the heat to a low and simmer, covered for about 30 minutes.

6. Meanwhile, in a skillet, heat the remaining oil over medium-high heat and cook the tempeh for about 3–5 minutes.

7. Stir in the dill and cook for about 1 minute.

8. Remove from the heat.

9. Remove the pan of soup from heat and stir in tomato paste and lemon juice.

10. With an immersion blender, blend the soup until smooth and creamy.

11. Serve the soup hot with the topping of tempeh.

Nutrition Info: Calories 294 Total Fat 15.7 g Saturated Fat 2.8 g Cholesterol 0 mg Sodium 723 mg Total Carbs 25.9 g Fiber 4.9 g Sugar 10.4 g Protein 16.4 g

Beet Soup

Servings: 2

Cooking Time: 5 Minutes

Ingredients:

- 2 cups coconut yogurt
- 4 teaspoons fresh lemon juice
- 2 cups beets, trimmed, peeled, and chopped
- 2 tablespoons fresh dill
- Salt, to taste
- 1 tablespoon pumpkin seeds
- 2 tablespoons coconut cream
- 1 tablespoon fresh chives, minced

Directions:

1. In a high-speed blender, add all ingredients and pulse until smooth.
2. Transfer the soup into a pan over medium heat and cook for about 3–5 minutes or until heated through.

3. Serve immediately with the garnishing of chives and coconut cream.

Nutrition Info: Calories 230 Total Fat 8 g Saturated Fat 5.8 g Cholesterol 0 mg Sodium 218 mg Total Carbs 33.5 g Fiber 4.2 g Sugar 27.5 g Protein 8 g

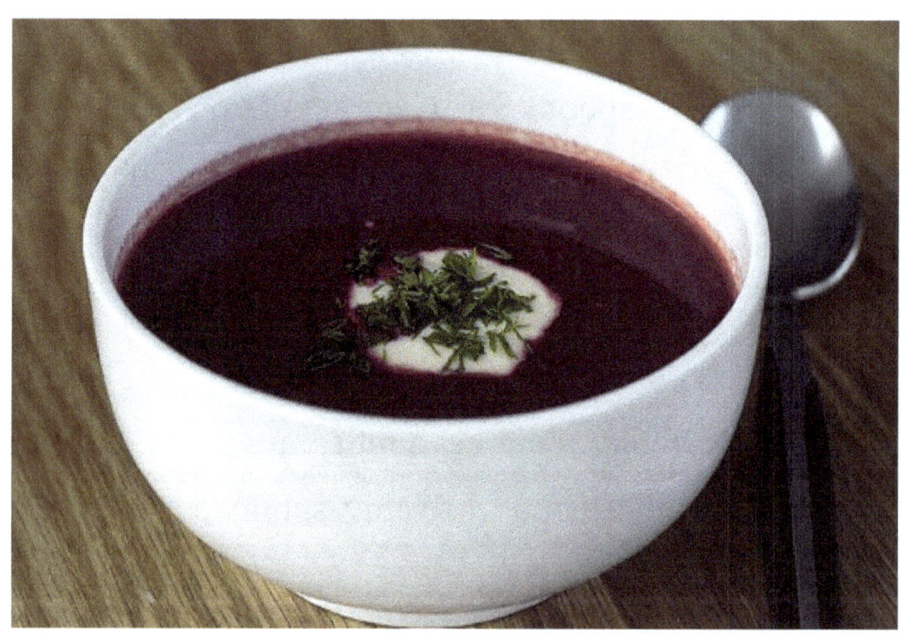

Balsamic Roasted Carrots

Servings: 4

Cooking Time: 30 Minutes

Ingredients:

- 1½ pounds carrots, quartered lengthwise
- 2 tablespoons extra-virgin olive oil
- ¼ teaspoon sea salt
- ⅛ teaspoon freshly ground black pepper
- 3 tablespoons balsamic vinegar

Directions:

1. Preheat the oven to 425°F.
2. In a large bowl, toss the carrots with the olive oil, sea salt, and pepper. Place in a single layer in a roasting pan or on a rimmed baking sheet. Roast for 20 to 30 minutes until the carrots are caramelized.
3. Toss with the vinegar and serve.

Nutrition Info: Calories: 132; Protein: 1g; Total Carbohydrates: 17g; Sugars: 8g; Fiber: 4g; Total Fat: 7g; Saturated Fat: 1g; Cholesterol: 0mg; Sodium: 235mg

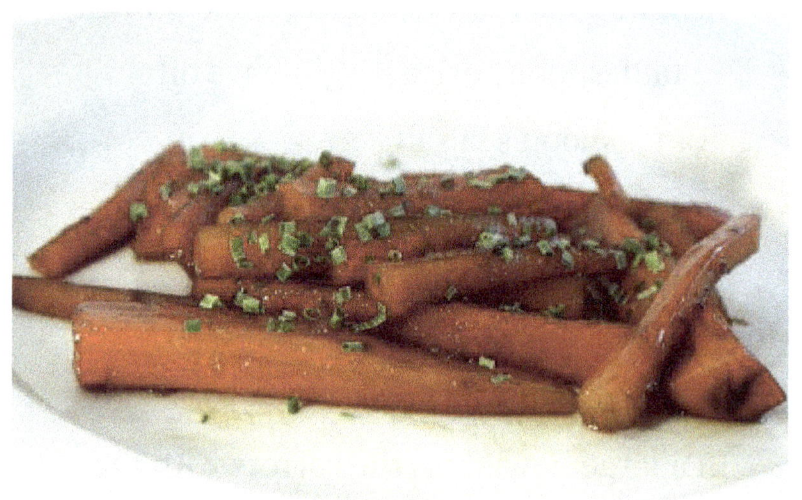

Roasted Lemon Mixed Vegetables

Servings: 5

Cooking Time: 20 Minutes

Ingredients:

- 2 teaspoons lemon zest
- 1-1/2 cups broccoli florets
- 1-1/2 cups cauliflower florets
- 1 teaspoon oregano, crushed
- ¾ cup red bell pepper, diced
- What you will need from the store cupboard:
- 1 tablespoon olive oil
- 2 sliced garlic cloves
- ¼ teaspoon salt

Directions:

1. Preheat your oven to 350 °F.
2. Bring together the broccoli, garlic, and cauliflower in a baking pan.
3. Drizzle oil. Sprinkle the salt and oregano.

4. Roast for 10 minutes.

5. Now add the bell pepper to the vegetables. Stir and combine.

6. Roast until the vegetables have become light brown and crisp.

7. Sprinkle lemon zest and serve.

Nutrition Info: Calories 52, Carbohydrates 5g, Fiber 2g, Cholesterol 0mg, Fat 3g, Sugar 0.2g, Protein 2g, Sodium 134mg

Butternut Fritters

Servings: 6

Cooking Time: 15 Minutes

Ingredients:

- 5 cup butternut squash, grated
- 2 large eggs
- 1 tablespoon. fresh sage, diced fine
- 2/3 cup flour
- 2 tablespoons olive oil
- Salt and pepper, to taste

Directions:

1. Heat oil in a large skillet over med-high heat.
2. In a large bowl, combine squash, eggs, sage and salt and pepper to taste. Fold in flour.
3. Drop ¼ cup mixture into skillet, keeping fritters at least 1 inch apart. Cook till golden brown on both sides, about 2 minutes per side.

4. Transfer to paper towel lined plate. Repeat. Serve immediately with your favorite dipping sauce.

Nutrition Info: Calories 164 Total Carbohydrates 24g Net Carbohydrates 21g Protein 4g Fat 6g Sugar 3g Fiber 3g

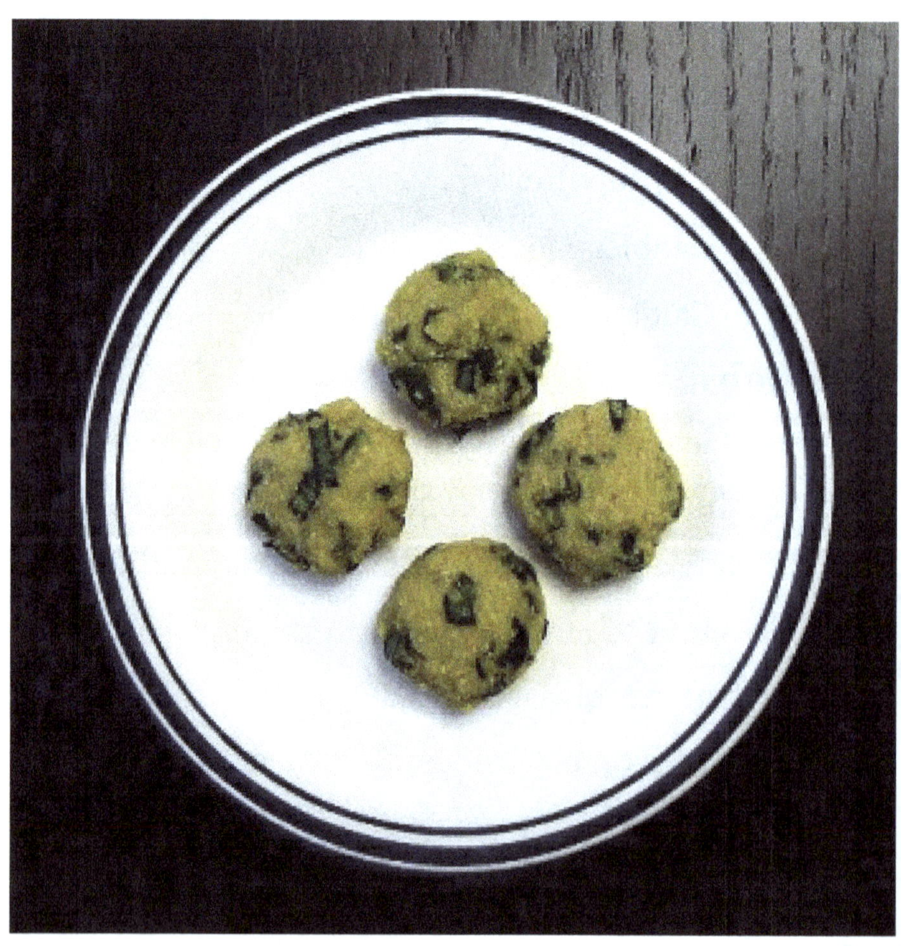

Mushroom Toast

Servings: 8

Cooking Time: 10 Minutes

Ingredients:

- 1 lb. button mushrooms

- 2 tablespoons thyme, chopped

- 3 tablespoons parsley, chopped

- 2 celery stalks, chopped

- 8 whole-grain bread slices, 1-inch slices

- What you will need from the store cupboard:

- 2 tablespoons sour cream, low-fat

- 1 crushed garlic clove

- ½ cup ricotta cheese

- Pinch of cayenne pepper

- Salt and pepper to taste

Directions:

1. Keep the celery, ricotta, cayenne pepper and parsley in a bowl. Mix well.

2. Preheat your oven to 350 °F.

3. Halve the large mushrooms. Place them in a big skillet.

4. Add the thyme, garlic, sour cream, and 1 teaspoon of water.

5. Cook covered until your mushrooms have become tender.

6. Season with pepper and salt.

7. In the meantime, toast both sides of the bread slices.

8. Apply ricotta mixture on one side of the toast. Cut it in half.

9. Place toasts on serving plates.

10. Now spoon the mushroom mixture over them before serving.

Nutrition Info: Calories 148, Carbohydrates 24g, Fiber 4g, Cholesterol 6mg, Sugar 0.3g, Fat 4g, Protein 8g

Cauliflower In Vegan Alfredo Sauce

Servings: 1

Cooking Time: 35 Minutes

Ingredients:

- Olive oil: 1 tablespoon
- Garlic: 2 cloves
- Vegetable broth: 1 cup
- Sea salt: ½ teaspoon
- Pepper: as per taste
- Chilli flakes: 1 teaspoon
- Onion (diced): 1 medium
- Cauliflower florets (chopped): 4 cups
- Lemon juice (freshly squeezed): 1 teaspoon
- nutritional yeast: 1 tablespoon
- Vegan butter: 2 tablespoons
- Zucchini noodles: for serving

Directions:

1. Begin by positioning a cooking pot on low heat. Stream in the oil and allow it to heat through.

2. Immediately you're done, toss in the chopped onion and set on fire for about 4 minutes. The onion should be translucent.

3. Put in the garlic and Prepare for about 30 seconds. Continuously stir to prevent them from sticking.

4. Put in the vegetable broth and shredded cauliflower florets. Ensure you mix well and cover the stockpot with a lid. Allow the cauliflower cook for 5 minutes and then extract it from the flame.

5. Get a blender and move the cooked cauliflower into it. Palpitate until the puree is smooth and creamy in texture. (Add 1 tablespoon of broth if required for.)

6. Put salt, lemon juice, nutritional yeast, butter, chilli flakes, and pepper to the

blender. Mix until all the ingredients fully combine to form a smooth puree.

7.   Position the zucchini noodles over a dishing platter and stream the Prepare cauliflower Alfredo sauce over the noodles.

Nutrition Info: Fat: 9.1 g Protein: 3.9 g Carbohydrates: 10 g

Citrus Sautéed Spinach

Servings: 4

Cooking Time: 5 Minutes

Ingredients:

- 2 tablespoons extra-virgin olive oil
- 4 cups fresh baby spinach
- 1 teaspoon orange zest
- ¼ cup freshly squeezed orange juice
- ½ teaspoon sea salt
- ⅛ teaspoon freshly ground black pepper

Directions:

1. In a large skillet over medium-high heat, heat the olive oil until it shimmers.
2. Add the spinach and orange zest. Cook for about 3 minutes, stirring occasionally, until the spinach wilts.
3. Stir in the orange juice, sea salt, and pepper. Cook for 2 minutes more, stirring occasionally. Serve hot.

Nutrition Info: Calories: 74; Protein: 7g; Total Carbohydrates: 3g; Sugars: 1g; Fiber: 1g; Total Fat: 7g; Saturated Fat: 1g;Cholesterol: 0mg;Sodium: 258mg

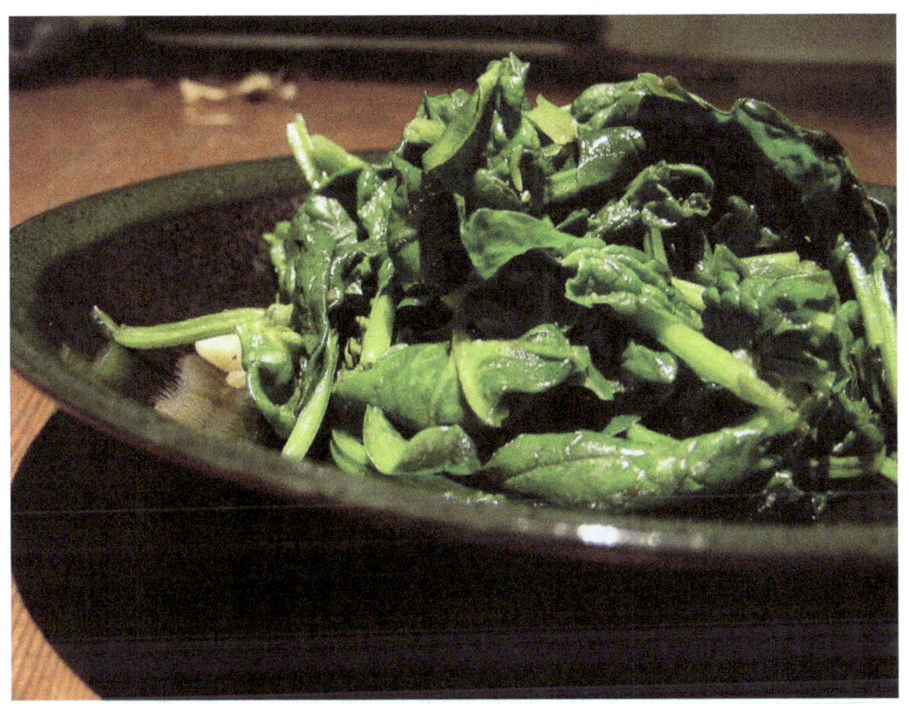

Tempeh With Bell Peppers

Servings: 3

Cooking Time: 15 Minutes

Ingredients:

- 2 tablespoons balsamic vinegar
- 2 tablespoons low-sodium soy sauce
- 2 tablespoons tomato sauce
- 1 teaspoon maple syrup
- ½ teaspoon garlic powder
- 1/8 teaspoon red pepper flakes, crushed
- 1 tablespoon vegetable oil
- 8 ounces' tempeh, cut into cubes
- 1 medium onion, chopped
- 2 large green bell peppers, seeded and chopped

Directions:

1. In a small bowl, add the vinegar, soy sauce, tomato sauce, maple syrup, garlic powder, and red pepper flakes and beat until well combined. Set aside.

2. Heat 1 tablespoon of oil in a large skillet over medium heat and cook the tempeh about 2–3 minutes per side.

3. Add the onion and bell peppers and heat for about 2–3 minutes.

4. Stir in the sauce mixture and cook for about 3–5 minutes, stirring frequently.

5. Serve hot.

Nutrition Info: Calories 241 Total Fat 13 g Saturated Fat 2.6 g Cholesterol 0 mg Sodium 65 mg Total Carbs 19.7 g Fiber 2.1 g Sugar 8.1 g Protein 16.1 g

Mushroom Curry

Servings: 3

Cooking Time: 20 Minutes

Ingredients:

- 2 cups tomatoes, chopped
- 1 green chili, chopped
- 1 teaspoon fresh ginger, chopped
- ¼ cup cashews
- 2 tablespoons canola oil
- ½ teaspoon cumin seeds
- ¼ teaspoon ground coriander
- ¼ teaspoon ground turmeric
- ¼ teaspoon red chili powder
- 1½ cups fresh shiitake mushrooms, sliced
- 1½ cups fresh button mushrooms, sliced
- 1 cup frozen corn kernels
- 1¼ cups water
- ¼ cup unsweetened coconut milk
- Salt and ground black pepper, to taste

Directions:

1. In a food processor, add the tomatoes, green chili, ginger, and cashews, and pulse until a smooth paste forms.
2. In a pan, heat the oil over medium heat and sauté the cumin seeds for about 1 minute.
3. Add the spices and sauté for about 1 minute.
4. Add the tomato paste and cook for about 5 minutes.
5. Stir in the mushrooms, corn, water, and coconut milk, and bring to a boil.
6. Cook for about 10–12 minutes, stirring occasionally.
7. Season with salt and black pepper and remove from the heat.
8. Serve hot.

Nutrition Info: Calories 311 Total Fat 20.4 g Saturated Fat 6.1 g Cholesterol 0 mg Sodium 244 mg Total Carbs 32g Fiber 5.6 g Sugar 9 g Protein 8 g

Bean Medley Chili

Servings: 8

Cooking Time: 20 Minutes

Ingredients:

- 1 can black beans, rinsed and drained
- 1 can garbanzo beans, rinsed and drained
- 1 teaspoon cumin, ground
- ¼ cup cilantro, snipped
- 2 onions, chopped
- What you will need from the store cupboard:
- 1 can chicken broth
- 3 tablespoons of chili powder
- 1 can chipotle chili pepper in adobo sauce
- ¼ teaspoon salt

Directions:

1. Bring together the beans, pepper, onion, chili powder, salt, and cumin in your cooker.
2. Add the broth.
3. Cover and cook.
4. Stir the cilantro in.
5. You can serve it with rice if desired.

Nutrition Info: Calories 191, Carbohydrates 38g, Cholesterol 0mg, Fiber 12g, Fat 2g, Protein 12g, Sugar 0.7g, Sodium 659mg

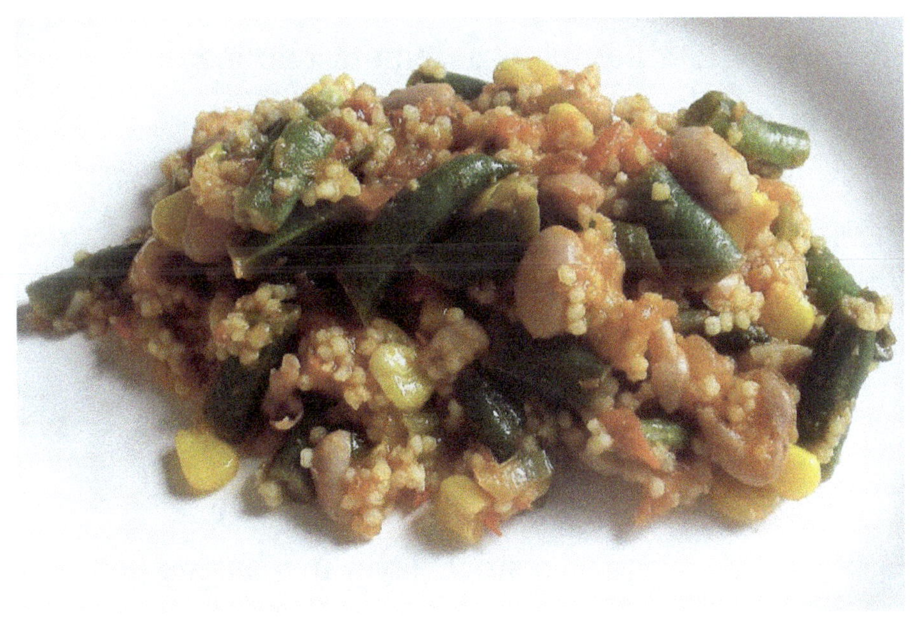

Roasted Carrots

Servings: 4

Cooking Time: 20 Minutes

Ingredients:

- 2 tablespoons olive oil, divided
- 2 tablespoons balsamic vinegar
- 1 tablespoon pure maple syrup
- 1 lb. carrots, sliced into small pieces
- Salt to taste
- 2 tablespoons hazelnuts, chopped

Directions:

1. Preheat your oven to 400 degrees F.
2. Combine 1 tablespoon oil with vinegar and maple syrup.
3. Set aside the mixture.
4. In another bowl, toss the carrots in remaining oil and season with salt.
5. Arrange on a single layer in a baking pan.
6. Roast for 15 minutes.

7. Pour the reserved mixture over the carrots and mix.

8. Roast for additional 5 minutes.

9. Sprinkle hazelnuts on top before serving.

Nutrition Info: Calories 130 Total Fat 7 g Saturated Fat 1g Cholesterol 0 mg Sodium 226 mg Total Carbohydrate 16 g Dietary Fiber 3 g Total Sugars 10 g Protein 1 g Potassium 382 mg

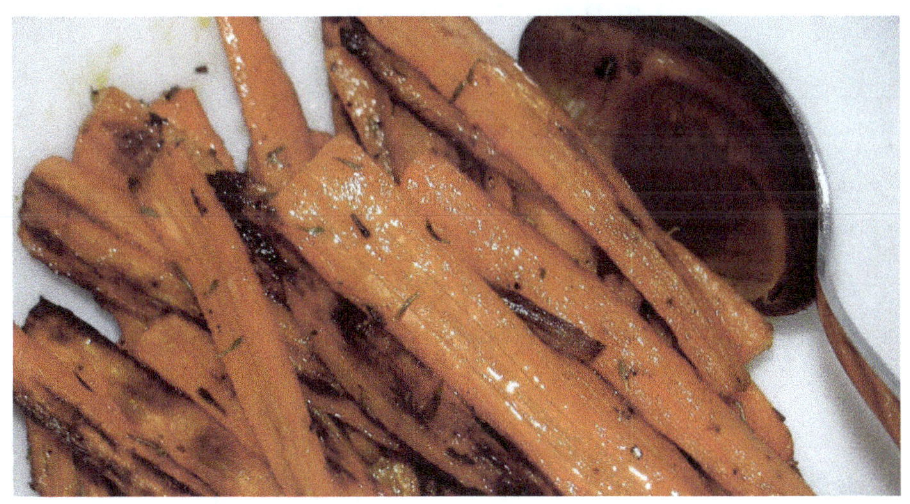

Boiled Potatoes With Tomato Salsa

Servings: 8

Cooking Time: 15 Minutes

Ingredients:

- 6 potatoes, sliced into wedges
- 1 clove garlic, minced
- 3 large tomatoes, diced
- 2 tablespoons white onion, chopped
- 2 teaspoons fresh marjoram, chopped
- Salt and pepper to taste

Directions:

1. Boil the potatoes until soft enough to poke with a fork.
2. Combine the rest of the ingredients in a bowl.
3. Serve potatoes with salsa.

Nutrition Info: Calories 200 Total Fat 10 g Saturated Fat 1 g Cholesterol 25 mg Sodium 81 mg Total Carbohydrate 10 g Dietary Fiber 5 g Total Sugars 1 g Protein 25 g Potassium 560 mg

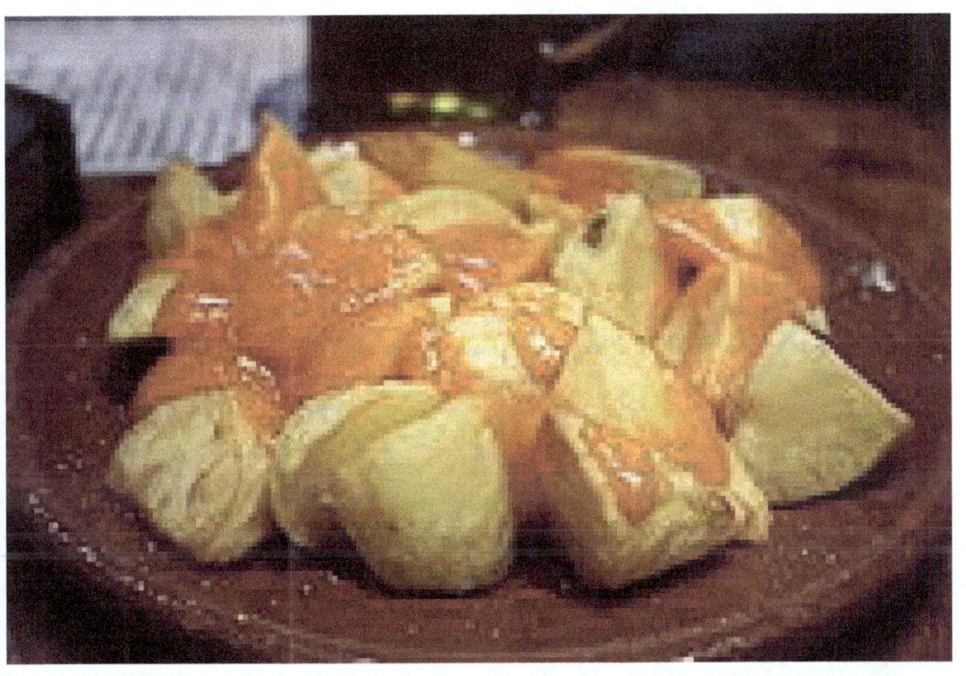

Lentil And Eggplant Stew

Servings: 2

Cooking Time: 35 Minutes

Ingredients:

- 1lb eggplant
- 1lb dry lentils
- 1 cup chopped vegetables
- 1 cup low sodium vegetable broth

Directions:

1. Mix all the ingredients in your Instant Pot.
2. Cook on Stew for 35 minutes.
3. Release the pressure naturally.

Nutrition Info: Calories: 310 Carbs: 22 Sugar: 6 Fat: 10 Protein: 32 GL: 16

Asian Fried Eggplant

Servings: 4

Cooking Time: 40 Minutes

Ingredients:

- 1 large eggplant, sliced into fourths
- 3 green onions, diced, green tips only
- 1 teaspoon fresh ginger, peeled & diced fine
- ¼ cup + 1 teaspoon cornstarch
- 1 ½ tablespoon. soy sauce
- 1 ½ tablespoon. sesame oil
- 1 tablespoon. vegetable oil
- 1 tablespoon. fish sauce
- 2 teaspoon Splenda
- ¼ teaspoon salt

Directions:

1. Place eggplant on paper towels and sprinkle both sides with salt. Let for 1 hour to remove excess moisture. Pat dry with more paper towels.

2. In a small bowl, whisk together soy sauce, sesame oil, fish sauce, Splenda, and 1 teaspoon cornstarch.

3. Coat both sides of the eggplant with the ¼ cup cornstarch, use more if needed.

4. Heat oil in a large skillet, over med-high heat. Add ½ the ginger and 1 green onion, then lay 2 slices of eggplant on top. Use ½ the sauce mixture to lightly coat both sides of the eggplant. Cook 8-10 minutes per side. Repeat.

5. Serve garnished with remaining green onions.

Nutrition Info: Calories 155 Total Carbohydrates 18g Net Carbohydrates 13g Protein 2g Fat 9g Sugar 6g Fiber 5g

Carrot Cake Bites

Servings: 22

Cooking Time: 15 Minutes

Ingredients:

- 4 oz. carrots, chopped
- ¼ cup chia seeds
- ¼ cup pecans, chopped
- ¼ teaspoon turmeric, ground
- ¾ teaspoon cinnamon, ground
- What you will need from the store cupboard:
- 1 teaspoon vanilla extract
- 1 cup pitted dates
- ¼ teaspoon salt
- Pinch of ground pepper

Directions:

1. Bring together the chia seeds, pecans, and dates in your food processor.

2. Pulse until everything is chopped and well combined.

3. Now add the vanilla, carrots, cinnamon, salt, pepper, and turmeric.

4. Process until you see a paste starting to form.

5. Create small balls by rolling this mixture.

Nutrition Info: Calories 48, Carbohydrates 8g, Fiber 2g, Cholesterol 0mg, Fat 2g, Sugar 0.5g, Protein 1g, Sodium 30mg

Broccoli With Ginger And Garlic

Servings: 4

Cooking Time: 11 Minutes

Ingredients:

- 2 tablespoons extra-virgin olive oil
- 2 cups broccoli florets
- 1 tablespoon grated fresh ginger
- ½ teaspoon sea salt
- ⅛ teaspoon freshly ground black pepper
- 3 garlic cloves, minced

Directions:

1. In a large skillet over medium-high heat, heat the olive oil until it shimmers.
2. Add the broccoli, ginger, sea salt, and pepper. Cook for about 10 minutes, stirring occasionally, until the broccoli is soft and starts to brown.

3. Add the garlic and cook for 30 seconds, stirring constantly. Remove from the heat and serve.

Nutrition Info: Per Serving Calories: 80; Protein: 1g; Total Carbohydrates: 4g; Sugars: 1g; Fiber: 1g; Total Fat: 0g; Saturated Fat: 1g; Cholesterol: 0mg; Sodium: 249mg

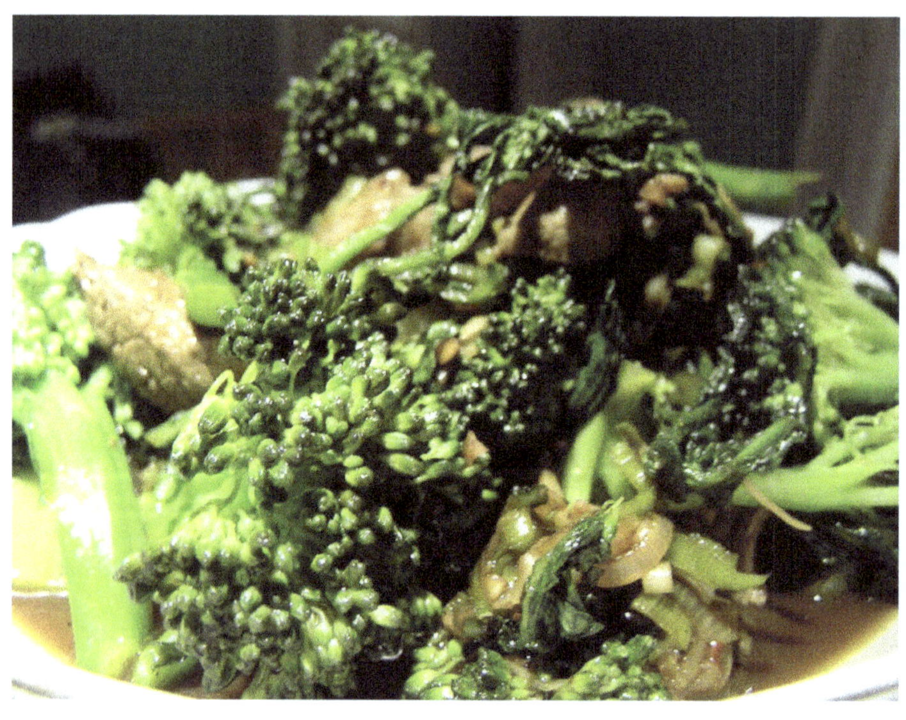

Barley Pilaf

Servings: 4

Cooking Time: 1 Hour 5 Minutes

Ingredients:

- ½ cup pearl barley
- 1 cup low-sodium vegetable broth
- 2 tablespoons olive oil, divided
- 2 garlic cloves, minced finely
- ½ cup onion, chopped
- ½ cup eggplant, sliced thinly
- ½ cup green bell pepper, seeded and chopped
- ½ cup red bell pepper, seeded and chopped
- 2 tablespoons fresh cilantro, chopped
- 2 tablespoons fresh mint leaves, chopped

Directions:

1. In a pan, add the barley and broth over medium-high heat and bring to a boil.

2. Immediately, reduce the heat to low and simmer, covered for about 45 minutes or until all the liquid is absorbed.

3. In a large skillet, heat 1 tablespoon of oil over high heat and sauté the garlic for about 1 minute.

4. Stir in the cooked barley and cook for about 3 minutes.

5. Remove from heat and set aside.

6. In another skillet, heat remaining oil over medium heat and sauté the onion for about 5-7 minutes.

7. Add the eggplant and bell peppers and stir fry for about 3 minutes.

8. Stir in the remaining ingredients except walnuts and cook for about 2-3 minutes.

9. Stir in barley mixture and cook for about 2-3 minutes.

10. Serve hot.

11. Meal Prep Tip: Transfer the pilaf into a large bowl and set aside to cool. Divide the pilaf into 4 containers evenly. Cover the containers

and refrigerate for 1 day. Reheat in the microwave before serving.

Nutrition Info: Calories 168 Total Fat 7.4 g Saturated Fat 1.1 g Cholesterol 0 mg Total Carbs 23.5 g Sugar 1.9 g Fiber 5 g Sodium 22 mg Potassium 164 mg Protein 3.6 g

Kale With Miso & Ginger

Servings: 6

Cooking Time: 10 Minutes

Ingredients:

- 8 oz. fresh kale, sliced into strips
- 1 clove garlic, minced
- 1 tablespoon lime juice
- ½ teaspoon lime zest
- 2 tablespoons oil
- 2 tablespoons rice vinegar
- 1 teaspoon fresh ginger, grated
- 2 teaspoons miso
- 2 tablespoons dry roasted cashews, chopped

Directions:

1. Steam kale on a steamer basket in a pot with water.
2. Transfer kale to a bowl.
3. Mix the rest of the ingredients except cashews in another bowl.
4. Toss kale in the mixture.
5. Top with chopped cashews before serving.

Nutrition Info: Calories 86 Total Fat 5 g Saturated Fat 0 g Cholesterol 0 mg Sodium 104 mg Total Carbohydrate 9 g Dietary Fiber 2 g Total Sugars 2 g Protein 3 g Potassium 352 mg

Beans, Walnuts & Veggie Burgers

Servings: 8

Cooking Time: 25 Minutes

Ingredients:

- ½ cup walnuts
- 1 carrot, peeled and chopped
- 1 celery stalk, chopped
- 4 scallions, chopped
- 5 garlic cloves, chopped
- 2¼ cups cooked black beans
- 2½ cups sweet potato, peeled and grated
- ½ teaspoon red pepper flakes, crushed
- ¼ teaspoon cayenne pepper
- Salt and ground black pepper, as required

Directions:

1. Preheat the oven to 400 degrees F. Line a baking sheet with parchment paper.
2. In a food processor, add walnuts and pulse until finely ground.
3. Add the carrot, celery, scallion and garlic and pulse until chopped finely.
4. Transfer the vegetable mixture into a large bowl.
5. In the same food processor, add beans and pulse until chopped.
6. Add 1½ cups of sweet potato and pulse until a chunky mixture forms.
7. Transfer the bean mixture into the bowl with vegetable mixture.
8. Stir in the remaining sweet potato and spices and mix until well combined.
9. Make 8 patties from mixture.
10. Arrange the patties onto prepared baking sheet in a single layer.
11. Bake for about 25 minutes.
12. Serve hot.

13. Meal Prep Tip: Remove the burgers from oven and set aside to cool completely. Store these burgers in an airtight container, by placing parchment papers between the burgers to avoid the sticking. These burgers can be stored in the freezer for up to 3 weeks. Before serving, thaw the burgers and then reheat in microwave.

Nutrition Info: Calories 177 Total Fat 5 g Saturated Fat 0.3 g Cholesterol 0 mg Total Carbs 27.6 g Sugar 5.3 g Fiber 7.6 g Sodium 205 mg Potassium 398 mg Protein 8 g

Artichoke Quiche

Servings: 6

Cooking Time: 15 Minutes

Ingredients:

- 2 cups long-grain rice, cooked
- ¾ cup egg substitute
- ¼ cup green onions, sliced
- ¼ teaspoon white pepper, ground
- 1 can artichoke hearts
- What you will need from the store cupboard:
- ¾ cup low-fat cheddar cheese
- 1 garlic clove, crushed
- ¾ cup fat-free milk
- ½ teaspoon salt
- 1 tablespoon Dijon mustard
- Cooking spray

Directions:

1.   Bring together the egg substitute, ¼ cup cheese, garlic, salt, and rice.
2.   Apply cooking spray to a pie plate. Bake for 5 minutes.
3.   Keep the artichoke quarters at the bottom of your rice crust.
4.   Now sprinkle the remaining cheese.
5.   Combine the remaining milk, egg substitute, and the other ingredients.
6.   Pour the cheese over.
7.   Bake until it sets.
8.   Cut into wedges and garnish with the onion strips.

Nutrition Info: Calories 169, Carbohydrates 23g, Fiber 1g, Cholesterol 11mg, Fat 4g, Protein 10g, Sodium 490mg

Quinoa In Tomato Sauce

Servings: 4

Cooking Time: 40 Minutes

Ingredients:

- 2 tablespoons olive oil
- 1 cup quinoa, rinsed
- 1 green bell pepper, seeded and chopped
- 1 medium onion, chopped finely
- 3 garlic cloves, minced
- 2½ cups filtered water
- 2 cups tomatoes, crushed finely
- 1 teaspoon red chili powder
- ¼ teaspoon ground cumin
- ¼ teaspoon garlic powder
- Ground black pepper, as required

Directions:

1. In a large pan, heat the oil over medium-high heat and cook the quinoa, onion, bell pepper and garlic for about 5 minutes, stirring frequently.
2. Stir in the remaining ingredients and bring to a boil.
3. Now, reduce the heat to medium-low.
4. Cover the pan tightly and simmer for about 30 minutes, stirring occasionally.
5. Serve hot.
6. Meal Prep Tip: Transfer the quinoa mixture into a large bowl and set aside to cool. Divide the chili into 4 containers evenly. Cover the containers and refrigerate for 1-2 days. Reheat in the microwave before serving.

Nutrition Info: Calories 260 Total Fat 10 g Saturated Fat 1.4 g Cholesterol 0 mg Total Carbs 36.9 g Sugar 5.2 g Fiber 5.4 g Sodium 16 mg Potassium 575 mg Protein 7.7 g

Black Bean With Poblano Tortilla Wraps

Servings: 4

Cooking Time: 10 Minutes

Ingredients:

- ½ teaspoon cumin, ground
- 1/3 cup poblano chili, chopped
- 1 cup avocado, diced and peeled
- ¼ cup red onion, chopped
- 1 can rinse and drained black beans
- What you will need from the store cupboard:
- ½ cup low-fat sour cream
- 3 tablespoons lime juice
- 4 flour tortillas
- ¼ teaspoon salt

Directions:

1. Combine the cumin and sour cream in a bowl. Use a whisk to stir.
2. Bring together the beans and other ingredients.
3. Spoon out the mixture at the center of the tortillas.
4. Roll them up. Cut through the middle.
5. Use wooden picks to secure.
6. Serve with your sour cream mixture.

Nutrition Info: Calories 298, Carbohydrates 40g, Fiber 5g, Cholesterol 16mg, Fat 13g, Protein 9g, Sodium 606mg

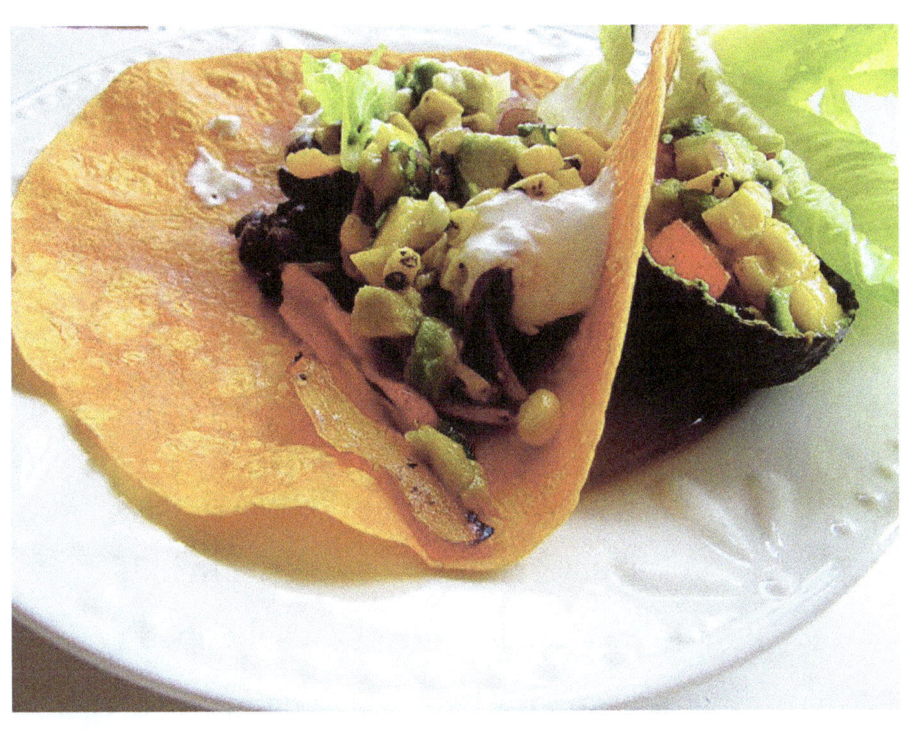

Mixed Greens Salad

Servings: 6

Cooking Time: 0 Minutes

Ingredients:

- 6 cups mixed salad greens
- 1 cup cucumber, chopped
- ½ cup carrot, shredded
- ¼ cup bell pepper, sliced into strips
- ¼ cup cherry tomatoes, sliced in half
- 6 tablespoons white onion, chopped
- 6 tablespoons balsamic vinaigrette dressing

Directions:

1. Toss all the ingredients in a large salad bowl.
2. Drizzle dressing on top or serve on the side.

Nutrition Info: Calories 23 Total Fat 1 g Saturated Fat 0 g Cholesterol 0 mg Sodium 138 mg Total Carbohydrate 4 g Dietary Fiber 1 g Total Sugars 1 g Protein 1 g Potassium 142 mg

Tofu Curry

Servings: 2

Cooking Time: 20 Minutes

Ingredients:

- 2 cups cubed extra firm tofu
- 2 cups mixed stir fry vegetables
- 0.5 cup soy yogurt
- 3tbsp curry paste
- 1tbsp oil or ghee

Directions:

1. Set the Instant Pot to saute and add the oil and curry paste.
2. When the onion is soft, add the remaining ingredients except the yogurt and seal.
3. Cook on Stew for 20 minutes.
4. Release the pressure naturally and serve with a scoop of soy yogurt.

Nutrition Info: Calories: 300 Carbs: 9 Sugar: 4 Fat: 14 Protein: 42 GL: 7

Baked Beans

Servings: 6

Cooking Time: 20 Minutes

Ingredients:

- 2 cups navy beans, overnight soaked in cold water
- 2/3 cups green bell pepper, diced
- 1 can tomatoes, diced
- 1 onion, sliced
- What you will need from the store cupboard:
- 3 tablespoons molasses
- ¼ cup of orange juice
- ¼ cup maple syrup
- 1 tablespoon Worcestershire sauce
- 1/4 teaspoon mustard powder
- 2 tablespoons stevia sugar
- 2 tablespoons salt

Directions:

1. Preheat your oven to 350 °F
2. Simmer the beans. Drain and keep the liquid.
3. Place beans in a casserole dish with the onion.
4. Bring together the dry mustard, pepper, salt, molasses, Worcestershire sauce, tomatoes, sugar substitute and orange juice in your saucepan.
5. Boil the mix. Pour over your beans.
6. Pour the reserved bean water, covering the beans.
7. Use aluminum foil to cover the dish.
8. Now bake in the oven. The beans must get tender.
9. Remove the foil and add some liquid if needed.

Nutrition Info: Calories 482, Carbohydrates 65g, Cholesterol 25mg, Fiber 12g, Fat 16g, Protein 21g, Sugar 2.2g, Sodium 512mg

Spicy Black Beans

Servings: 6

Cooking Time: 1½ Hours

Ingredients:

- 4 cups filtered water
- 1½ cups dried black beans, soaked for 8 hours and drained
- ½ teaspoon ground turmeric
- 3 tablespoons olive oil
- 1 small onion, chopped finely
- 1 green chili, chopped
- 1 (1-inch) piece fresh ginger, minced
- 2 garlic cloves, minced
- 1-1½ tablespoons ground coriander
- 1 teaspoon ground cumin
- ½ teaspoon cayenne pepper
- Sea salt, as required
- 2 medium tomatoes, chopped finely
- ½ cup fresh cilantro, chopped

Directions:

1. In a large pan, add water, black beans and turmeric and bring to a boil on high heat.
2. Now, reduce the heat to low and simmer, covered for about 1 hour or till desired doneness of beans.
3. Meanwhile, in a skillet, heat the oil over medium heat and sauté the onion for about 4-5 minutes.
4. Add the green chili, ginger, garlic, spices and salt and sauté for about 1-2 minutes.
5. Stir in the tomatoes and cook for about 10 minutes, stirring occasionally.
6. Transfer the tomato mixture into the pan with black beans and stir to combine.
7. Increase the heat to medium-low and simmer for about 15-20 minutes.
8. Stir in the cilantro and simmer for about 5 minutes.
9. Serve hot.
10. Meal Prep Tip: Transfer the beans mixture into a large bowl and set aside to cool. Divide

the mixture into 6 containers evenly. Cover
the containers and refrigerate for 1-2 days.
Reheat in the microwave before serving.

Nutrition Info: Calories 160 Total Fat 8 g Saturated
Fat 1 g Cholesterol 0 mg Total Carbs 17.9 g Sugar 2.4 g
Fiber 6.2 g Sodium 50 mg Potassium 343 mg Protein 6
g

Cauliflower Mushroom Risotto

Servings: 2

Cooking Time: 30 Minutes

Ingredients:

- 1 medium head cauliflower, grated
- 8-ounce Porcini mushrooms, sliced
- 1 yellow onion, diced fine
- 2 cup low sodium vegetable broth
- 2 teaspoon garlic, diced fine
- 2 teaspoon white wine vinegar
- Salt & pepper, to taste
- Olive oil cooking spray

Directions:

1. Heat oven to 350 degrees. Line a baking sheet with foil.

2. Place the mushrooms on the prepared pan and spray with cooking spray. Sprinkle with salt and toss to coat. Bake 10-12 minutes, or

until golden brown and the mushrooms start to crisp.

3. Spray a large skillet with cooking spray and place over med-high heat. Add onion and cook, stirring frequently, until translucent, about 3-4 minutes. Add garlic and cook 2 minutes, until golden.

4. Add the cauliflower and cook 1 minute, stirring.

5. Place the broth in a saucepan and bring to a simmer. Add to the skillet, ¼ cup at a time, mixing well after each addition.

6. Stir in vinegar. Reduce heat to low and let simmer, 4-5 minutes, or until most of the liquid has evaporated.

7. Spoon cauliflower mixture onto plates, or in bowls, and top with mushrooms. Serve.

Nutrition Info: Calories 134 Total Carbohydrates 22g Protein 10g Fat 0g Sugar 5g Fiber 2g

Tofu With Peas

Servings: 5

Cooking Time: 20 Minutes

Ingredients:

- 1 tablespoon chili-garlic sauce
- 3 tablespoons low-sodium soy sauce
- 2 tablespoons canola oil, divided
- 1 (16-ounce) package extra-firm tofu, drained, pressed, and cubed
- 1 cup yellow onion, chopped
- 1 tablespoon fresh ginger, minced
- 2 garlic cloves, minced
- 2 large tomatoes, chopped finely
- 5 cups frozen peas, thawed
- 1 teaspoon white sesame seeds

Directions:

1. For sauce: in a bowl, add the chili-garlic sauce and soy sauce and mix until well combined.

2. In a large skillet, heat 1 tablespoon of oil over medium-high heat and cook the tofu for about 4–5 minutes or until browned completely, stirring occasionally.

3. Transfer the tofu into a bowl.

4. In the same skillet, heat the remaining oil over medium heat and sauté the onion for about 3–4 minutes.

5. Add the ginger and garlic and sauté for about 1 minute.

6. Add the tomatoes and cook for about 4–5 minutes, crushing with the back of spoon.

7. Stir in all three peas and cook for about 2–3 minutes.

8. Stir in the sauce mixture and tofu and cook for about 1–2 minutes.

9. Serve hot with the garnishing of sesame seeds.

Nutrition Info: Calories 291 Total Fat 11.9 g Saturated Fat 1.1 g Cholesterol 0 mg Sodium 732 mg Total Carbs 31.6 g Fiber 10.8 g Sugar 11.5 g Protein 19 g

Cauliflower And Kabocha Squash Soup

Servings: 1

Cooking Time: 35 Minutes

Ingredients:

- Olive oil: 2 tablespoons
- Garlic (minced): 3 cloves
- Cauliflower florets: 2½ cups
- Ground cardamom: ½ teaspoon
- Bay leaves: 2
- Vanilla almond milk (unsweetened): ½ cup
- Pepper: ¼ teaspoon
- Yellow onion (diced): ½
- Fresh ginger (minced): 1 tablespoon
- Kabocha squash (cubed): 2½ cups
- Cayenne: ¼ teaspoon
- Vegetable broth: 4 cups
- Salt: ½ teaspoon

Directions:

1. Begin by streaming the olive oil into a nonstick saucepan and position it over a high flame.
2. Toss in the onion, ginger, and garlic. Sauté for around 3 minutes.
3. Then put in the squash, cauliflower, cayenne, bay leaves, and cardamom. Combine well.
4. Stream in the vegetable broth and take the vegetables and stock mixture to a boil.
5. Reduce the flame and allow the soup simmer for 10 minutes.
6. Extract the pan and use the blender to puree the mixture.
7. Immediately the soup is pureed, replace the pan to the low heat. Put in the almond milk. Combine well.
8. Finalize by spicing with pepper and salt.

Nutrition Info: Fat: 7.7 g Protein: 3.4 g Carbohydrates: 11.6 g

Mango Tofu Curry

Servings: 2

Cooking Time: 35 Minutes

Ingredients:

- 1lb cubed extra firm tofu
- 1lb chopped vegetables
- 1 cup low carb mango sauce
- 1 cup vegetable broth
- 2tbsp curry paste

Directions:

1. Mix all the ingredients in your Instant Pot.
2. Cook on Stew for 35 minutes.
3. Release the pressure naturally.

Nutrition Info: Calories: 310 Carbs: 20 Sugar: 9 Fat: 4 Protein: 37 GL: 19

Banana Curry

Servings: 3

Cooking Time: 15 Minutes

Ingredients:

- 2 tablespoons olive
- 2 yellow onions, chopped
- 8 garlic cloves, minced
- 2 tablespoons curry powder
- 1 tablespoon ground ginger
- 1 tablespoon ground cumin
- 1 teaspoon ground turmeric
- 1 teaspoon ground cinnamon
- 1 teaspoon red chili powder
- Salt and ground black pepper, to taste
- 2/3 cup soy yogurt
- 1 cup tomato puree
- 2 bananas, peeled and sliced
- 3 tomatoes, chopped finely
- ¼ cup unsweetened coconut flakes

Directions:

1. In a large pan, heat the oil over medium heat and sauté onion for about 4–5 minutes.
2. Add the garlic, curry powder, and spices, and sauté for about 1 minute.
3. Add the soy yogurt and tomato sauce and bring to a gentle boil.
4. Stir in the bananas and simmer for about 3 minutes.
5. Stir in the tomatoes and simmer for about 1–2 minutes.
6. Stir in the coconut flakes and immediately remove from the heat.
7. Serve hot.

Nutrition Info: Calories 382 Total Fat 18.2 g Saturated Fat 6.6 g Cholesterol 0 mg Sodium 108 mg Total Carbs 53.4 g Fiber 11.3 g Sugar 24.8 g Protein 9 g

Dried Fruit Squash

Servings: 4

Cooking Time: 40 Minutes

Ingredients:

- ¼ cup water
- 1 medium butternut squash, halved and seeded
- ½ tablespoon olive oil
- ½ tablespoon balsamic vinegar
- Salt and ground black pepper, to taste
- 4 large dates, pitted and chopped
- 4 fresh figs, chopped
- 3 tablespoons pistachios, chopped
- 2 tablespoons pumpkin seeds

Directions:

1. Preheat the oven to 375°F.
2. Place the water in the bottom of a baking dish.

3. Arrange the squash halves in a large baking dish, hollow-side up, and drizzle with oil and vinegar.
4. Sprinkle with salt and black pepper.
5. Spread the dates, figs, and pistachios on top.
6. Bake for about 40 minutes, or until squash becomes tender.
7. Serve hot with the garnishing of pumpkin seeds.

Nutrition Info: Calories 227 Total Fat 5.5 g Saturated Fat 0.8 g Cholesterol 0 mg Sodium 66 mg Total Carbs 46.4 g Fiber 7.5 g Sugar 19.6 g Protein 5 g

Fake On-stew

Servings: 2

Cooking Time: 25 Minutes

Ingredients:

- 0.5lb soy bacon
- 1lb chopped vegetables
- 1 cup low sodium vegetable broth
- 1tbsp nutritional yeast

Directions:

1. Mix all the ingredients in your Instant Pot.
2. Cook on Stew for 25 minutes.
3. Release the pressure naturally.

Nutrition Info: Calories: 200 Carbs: 12 Sugar: 3 Fat: 7 Protein: 41 GL: 5

Squash Medley

Servings: 2

Cooking Time: 20 Minutes.

Ingredients:

- 2lbs mixed squash
- 0.5 cup mixed veg
- 1 cup vegetable stock
- 2tbsp olive oil
- 2tbsp mixed herbs

Directions:

1. Put the squash in the steamer basket and add the stock into the Instant Pot.
2. Steam the squash in your Instant Pot for 10 minutes.
3. Depressurize and pour away the remaining stock.
4. Set to saute and add the oil and remaining ingredients.
5. Cook until a light crust forms.

Nutrition Info: Calories: 100 Carbs: 10 Sugar: 3 Fat: 6 Protein: 5 GL: 20

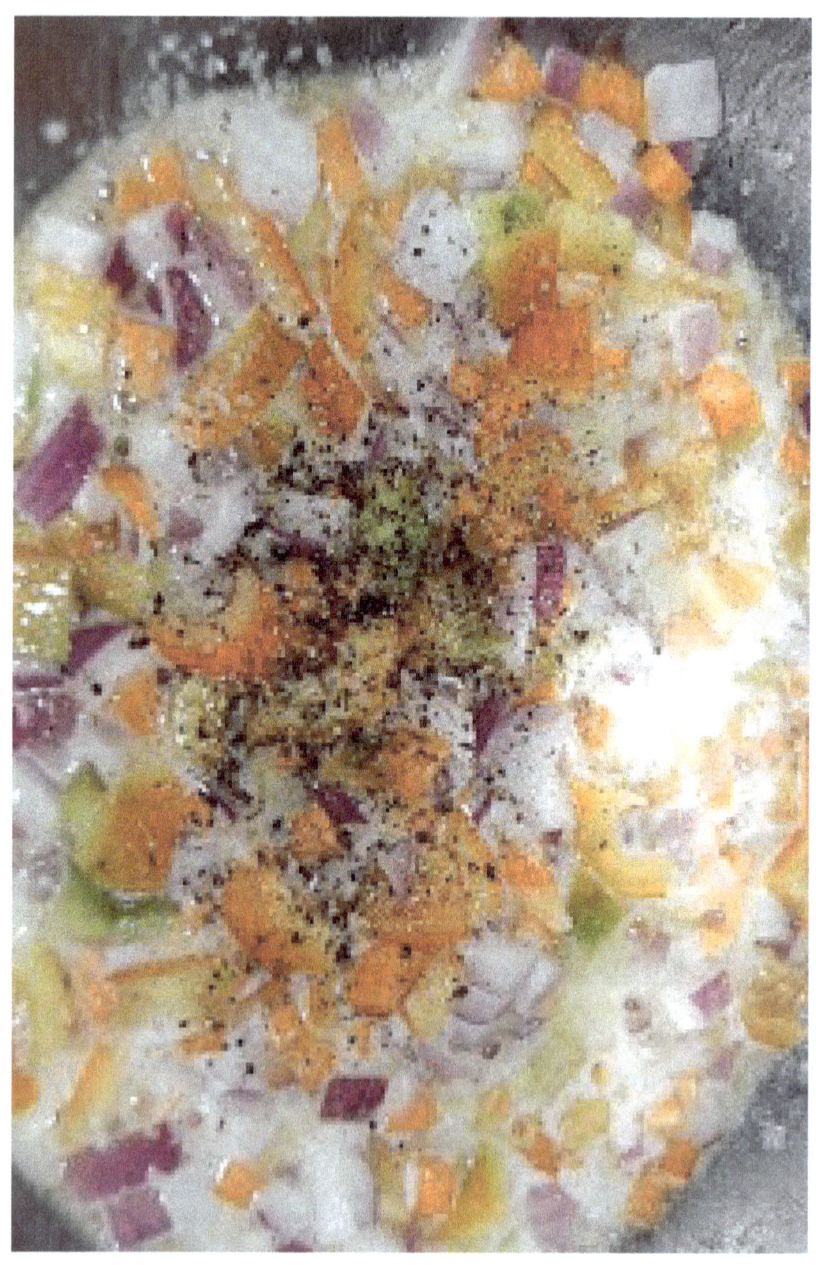

Porcini Mushrooms & Eggplant

Servings: 6

Cooking Time: 30 Minutes

Ingredients:

- 1 lb. eggplant, cubed
- 2 tablespoons olive oil
- Salt and pepper to taste
- ½ oz. dried porcini mushrooms
- 1 cup boiling water
- ⅓ cup balsamic vinegar
- 1 teaspoon fresh thyme, chopped
- ½ cup cherry tomatoes, sliced in half
- 1 tablespoon fresh basil, chopped

Directions:

1. Preheat your oven to 425 degrees F.
2. Arrange the eggplant cubes on a baking pan.
3. Drizzle oil on top and season with salt and pepper.
4. Roast for 15 minutes.

5. While waiting, soak mushrooms in hot water.

6. Let it sit for 15 minutes.

7. Drain water, and then chop.

8. Pour the vinegar in a saucepan over medium heat.

9. Bring to a boil and then reduce heat to simmer for 5 minutes.

10. Add the mushrooms and fresh thyme.

11. Drizzle balsamic mixture on top of the eggplants and serve with the tomatoes with basil.

Nutrition Info: Calories 77 Total Fat 5 g Saturated Fat 1 g Cholesterol 0 mg Sodium 103 mg Total Carbohydrate 8 g Dietary Fiber 3 g Total Sugars 4 g Protein 1 g Potassium 232 mg

Roasted Asparagus With Lemon And Pine Nuts

Servings: 4

Cooking Time: 20 Minutes

Ingredients:

- 1-pound asparagus, trimmed
- 2 tablespoons extra-virgin olive oil
- Juice of 1 lemon
- Zest of 1 lemon
- ¼ cup pine nuts
- ½ teaspoon sea salt
- ⅛ teaspoon freshly ground black pepper

Directions:

1. Preheat the oven to 425°F.
2. In a large bowl, toss the asparagus with the olive oil, lemon juice and zest, pine nuts, sea salt, and pepper. Spread in a roasting pan in an even layer.

3. Roast for about 20 minutes until the asparagus is browned.

Nutrition Info: Calories: 144; Protein: 4g; Total Carbohydrates: 6g; Sugars: 3g; Fiber: 3g; Total Fat: 13g;Saturated Fat: 1g; Cholesterol: 0mg; Sodium: 240mg

Veggie Stew

Servings: 3

Cooking Time: 30 Minutes

Ingredients:

- 2 tablespoons olive oil
- 1 large onion, chopped
- 2 garlic cloves, minced
- ¼ teaspoon fresh ginger, grated finely
- 1 teaspoon ground cumin
- 1 teaspoon cayenne pepper
- Salt and ground black pepper, to taste
- 2 cups homemade vegetable broth
- 1½ cups small broccoli florets
- 1½ cups small cauliflower florets
- 1 tablespoon fresh lemon juice
- 1 cup cashews
- 1 teaspoon fresh lemon zest, grated finely

Directions:

1. In a large soup pan, heat oil over medium heat and sauté the onion for about 3–4 minutes.
2. Add the garlic, ginger, and spices and sauté for about 1 minute.
3. Add 1 cup of the broth and bring to a boil.
4. Add the vegetables and again bring to a boil.
5. Cover the soup pan and cook for about 15–20 minutes, stirring occasionally.
6. Stir in the lemon juice and remove from the heat.
7. Serve hot with the topping of cashews and lemon zest.

Nutrition Info: Calories 425 Total Fat 32 g Saturated Fat 5.9 g Cholesterol 0 mg Sodium 601 mg Total Carbs 27.6 g Fiber 5.2 g Sugar 7.1 g Protein 13.4 g

Spiced Couscous Tomatoes

Servings: 8

Cooking Time: 15 Minutes

Ingredients:

- ½ teaspoon cumin, ground
- 1 teaspoon coriander, ground
- 8 beefsteak tomatoes
- ½ cup sliced almonds
- 1 eggplant, cut into ½ inch slices
- What you will need from the store cupboard:
- 1 cup vegetable broth, low-sodium
- 1 tablespoon olive oil
- ½ cup couscous
- 1 teaspoon harissa paste
- Salt and pepper to taste
- Pinch of ground cinnamon

Directions:

1. Sprinkle some salt inside the hollowed-out tomatoes.
2. Keep them on a plate, upside down. Use paper towels to cover.
3. Heat ½ of the olive oil in your saucepan.
4. Add almonds. Cook for 2-3 minutes over low temperature.
5. Add the other ingredients to the saucepan.
6. Stir the eggplant in. Cook while turning until it is tender and brown.
7. Stir in the cumin, cinnamon, and coriander.
8. Pour the broth in and boil. Now add the couscous.
9. Take out from the heat. Keep aside for 5 minutes.
10. Return to low temperature. Cook for 2 minutes.
11. Use a fork, separating the couscous grains.
12. Stir the almonds in and add the harissa paste to the mix.

13. Pour over the couscous. Season with pepper.
   Mix well.

14. Spoon the mixture into your tomatoes.

Nutrition Info: Calories 175, Fat 6g, Protein 5g, Carbohydrates 28g, Fiber 5g, Cholesterol 0mg, Sugar 1.1g

Black Bean And Veggie Soup Topped With Lime Salsa

Servings: 1

Cooking Time: 35 Minutes

Ingredients:

- Onions (diced): 2
- Celery (diced): 3 sticks
- Garlic (finely chopped): 3 cloves
- Cilantro: ½ bunch
- Dried oregano: 1 tablespoon
- Sea salt: ½ tablespoon
- Boiling water: 1 quart
- Salad onion (finely chopped): ½ small
- Carrots (diced): 2
- Red bell peppers (diced): 2
- Red chilis (remove seed): 2
- Bay leaf: 1
- Black pepper (freshly ground): 1 tablespoon

- Black beans (drained and rinsed): 2 cans (15 ounces)

- Tomato (finely chopped): 1

- Fresh juice of ½ lime

Directions:

1. Begin by extracting the leaves and stalks from the cilantro. Neatly shred the stalks and leaves. Arrange aside

2. Ge a large saucepan and stream in 3 tablespoons of water. In this, put the carrots, onions, bell peppers, celery, red chillies, garlic, coriander stalks, oregano, bay leaf, sea salt, and pepper. Mix until well-combined. Cover the pan using a lid and allow the veggies to cook for about 10 minutes. Keep mixing.

3. Put the black beans and boiling water into the saucepan. Keep stirring.

4. Extract the lid from the saucepan and low heat. Allow the soup to cook for half a minute.

5. While the soup is on a high flame, form the lime salsa. In this, you will mix the tomato,

salad onion, and cilantro leaves in a small bowl. Crush in the fresh lime juice.

6.   Stream the soup in a big and deep bowl and finish by topping with lime salsa.

Nutrition Info: Fat: 2.4 g Protein: 17.2 g Carbohydrates: 53.9 g

Chili Sin Carne

Servings: 2

Cooking Time: 35 Minutes

Ingredients:

- 3 cups mixed cooked beans
- 2 cups chopped tomatoes
- 1tbsp yeast extract
- 2 squares very dark chocolate
- 1tbsp red chili flakes

Directions:

1. Mix all the ingredients in your Instant Pot.
2. Cook on Beans for 35 minutes.
3. Release the pressure naturally.

Nutrition Info: Calories: 240 Carbs: 20 Sugar: 5 Fat: 3 Protein: 36 GL: 11

3-veggie Combo

Servings: 4

Cooking Time: 25 Minutes

Ingredients:

- 1 tablespoon olive oil
- 1 small yellow onion, chopped
- 1 teaspoon fresh thyme, chopped
- 1 garlic clove, minced
- 8 ounces' fresh button mushroom, sliced
- 1 pound Brussels sprouts
- 3 cups fresh spinach
- 4 tablespoons walnuts
- Salt and ground black pepper, to taste

Directions:

1. In a large skillet, heat the oil over medium heat and sauté the onion for about 3–4 minutes.

2. Add the thyme and garlic and sauté for about 1 minute.

3. Add the mushrooms and cook for about 15 minutes, or until caramelized.
4. Add the Brussels sprouts and cook for about 2–3 minutes.
5. Stir in the spinach and cook for about 3–4 minutes.
6. Stir in the walnuts, salt, and black pepper, and remove from the heat.
7. Serve hot.

Nutrition Info: Calories 153 Total Fat 8.8 g Saturated Fat 0.9 g Cholesterol 0 mg Sodium 94 mg Total Carbs 15.8 g Fiber 6.3 g Sugar 4.4 g Protein 8.5 g

Lentil And Chickpea Curry

Servings: 2

Cooking Time: 20 Minutes

Ingredients:

- 2 cups dry lentils and chickpeas
- 1 thinly sliced onion
- 1 cup chopped tomato
- 3tbsp curry paste
- 1tbsp oil or ghee

Directions:

1. Set the Instant Pot to saute and add the onion, oil, and curry paste.
2. When the onion is soft, add the remaining ingredients and seal.
3. Cook on Stew for 20 minutes.
4. Release the pressure naturally.

Nutrition Info: Calories: 360 Carbs: 26 Sugar: 6 Fat: 19 Protein: 23 GL: 10